# OVERCOME PERIPHERAL ARTERY DISEASE

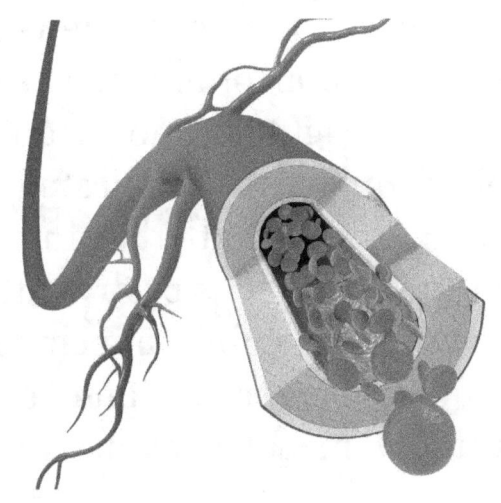

## Taking Charge of Your Health A Roadmap to Managing Peripheral Artery Disease

## Dr.Rebecca J. Reynolds

# Foreword

Welcome to the inspiring journey of "Overcome Peripheral Artery Disease." This book serves as a beacon of hope and knowledge for those facing the challenges of this often underestimated condition. As someone who has witnessed the resilience of individuals confronting Peripheral Artery Disease (PAD), I am deeply honored to introduce you to this invaluable resource.

Peripheral Artery Disease is a formidable adversary, affecting millions of lives worldwide. It's a condition that can quietly creep into our bodies, limiting our mobility, causing discomfort, and posing serious health risks. But within the pages of this book, you will discover that PAD is not invincible. With determination, understanding, and the right guidance, you can take significant steps toward regaining control of your life.

# Dear Buyers of "Overcome Peripheral Artery Disease,"

We want you to know that this book was written with a singular mission – to bring back smiles to the faces of all those who are suffering from the bondage of Peripheral Artery Disease (PAD). We understand the challenges and uncertainties that come with this condition, but we firmly believe in the power of knowledge, resilience, and hope.

In the pages of this book, you will find a wealth of information, practical advice, and inspirational stories that aim to uplift your spirits and guide you towards a brighter future. We want you to know that you are not alone on this journey. Many have walked the path you're on, and their triumphs serve as a beacon of hope for you.

Our goal is to empower you with knowledge, equip you with strategies to manage PAD effectively, and inspire you to face each day with renewed determination. We want to see those smiles return, the joy resurface, and the quality of life improve.

So, as you embark on this journey with "Overcome Peripheral Artery Disease," remember that there is a community of support within these pages, and you have the strength within you to overcome the challenges that PAD presents. Together, we aim to bring back those smiles and create a brighter, healthier tomorrow.

# CONTENT

# INTRODUCTION

Welcome to "Overcome Peripheral Artery Disease," a comprehensive guide dedicated to empowering you on your journey to conquer this challenging condition and regain control over your life. Peripheral Artery Disease, often abbreviated as PAD, affects millions of individuals around the world, and we understand that facing it can be daunting.

In the pages of this book, we have crafted a roadmap that will walk you through understanding the intricacies of PAD, exploring the latest advancements in diagnosis and treatment, and providing you with practical strategies to not just manage but overcome this condition.

We believe that knowledge is a powerful tool, and as you delve into these chapters, you'll gain insights into the underlying causes, symptoms, and risk factors associated with PAD. But this guide goes beyond the basics. We delve into lifestyle modifications, medications, surgical options, and innovative therapies that can significantly improve your quality of life.

Moreover, we recognize that living with PAD extends beyond the physical realm. This book offers guidance on maintaining emotional well-being, building a strong support network, and staying motivated throughout your journey.

We've also gathered inspirational stories from individuals who have successfully overcome PAD, proving that a fulfilling life is within reach.

Whether you're a newly diagnosed patient or someone who has been dealing with PAD for years, this book is your companion in the fight against peripheral artery disease. It is our hope that you'll find the information, resources, and encouragement you need to not just manage but triumph over PAD and build a healthier, more vibrant future. Your journey begins now

# Real-life Triumphs Over PAD

Once upon a time in a quiet suburban neighborhood, there lived a man named William. He was known for his cheerful demeanor and active lifestyle. He loved to take long walks around his picturesque community, admiring the blooming flowers and chatting with his neighbors.

However, as the years went by, William began to notice a change in his ability to walk. He'd experience painful cramps in his legs, especially during his walks, and his once-frequent strolls became shorter and more infrequent. Even worse, his feet would often feel cold and tingly.

Concerned about his health, William decided to consult his doctor. After a series of tests and examinations, he was diagnosed with Peripheral Artery Disease (PAD). His doctor explained that PAD was a condition in which narrowed arteries reduced blood flow to his legs, causing the discomfort and cramping he had been experiencing.

William was initially disheartened by the diagnosis, fearing that his active lifestyle was now a thing of the past. However, his doctor reassured him that with the right approach, he could manage his PAD effectively.

Determined not to let PAD control his life, William embarked on a journey of lifestyle changes. He started a structured exercise program recommended by his healthcare provider, which included walking sessions designed to improve his circulation. He also adjusted his diet to include heart-healthy foods and quit smoking, a habit he had held onto for far too long.

Over time, William noticed a gradual improvement in his symptoms. His walks became longer, and he experienced fewer cramps and discomfort. He even joined a local PAD support group, where he met others facing similar challenges, and their shared experiences provided him with inspiration and motivation.

With dedication and support, William's quality of life began to improve. He may not have been able to walk as far or as fast as he used to, but he found joy in each step he took. His neighborhood walks became an opportunity to appreciate the beauty around him and share a smile and a friendly chat with his neighbors.

William's story serves as a reminder that even in the face of challenges like PAD, determination, lifestyle changes, and a supportive community can help individuals regain their vitality and continue to find happiness in life's simple pleasures.

# Chapter 1

## Unveiling Peripheral Artery Disease

## Peripheral artery disease: what is it

A buildup of plaque in the arteries in your legs is called peripheral artery disease (PAD).
The blood that flows from your heart to your arms and legs is enriched with nutrients and oxygen thanks to the leg arteries.
Peripheral arterial disease and peripheral vascular disease are additional names for this condition.

A smooth inner surface on the inside of the hollow tubes-like arteries keeps blood from clotting and encourages constant blood flow.

Plaque, which is composed of fat, cholesterol, and other substances, gradually develops inside the walls of your arteries when you have peripheral artery disease.
This gradually narrows your arteries.
Atherosclerosis is another name for this plaque.

Many plaque deposits have a hard exterior and a soft interior.
In order to help your blood clot, platelets, which are shaped like discs, can travel to the area when the hard surface cracks or tears.
If blood clots develop around the plaque, your artery will become even more constricted.

Your arteries become narrowed or blocked by plaque or blood clots, making it difficult for blood to reach your organs and other tissues.
This harms the tissues beneath the blockage, leading to eventual death (gangrene).
Your feet and toes are where this occurs the most frequently.

In some people more than others, PAD can deteriorate more quickly.

Where the plaque develops on your body and your general health are two additional factors that are important.

## What effects will peripheral artery disease have on my body

Claudication, a medical term for leg pain that begins during exercise or walking and subsides with rest, is a typical symptom of PAD.
Your leg muscles are suffering because they aren't receiving enough oxygen.

The risks associated with PAD go far beyond issues with walking.
A non-healing sore on your legs or feet is more likely if you have peripheral artery disease.
These sores can develop into areas of dead tissue (gangrene) in cases of severe PAD, necessitating the removal of your foot or leg.

# What phases of peripheral artery disease are there

Fontaine and Rutherford are two different systems that healthcare providers can use to categorize your PAD.
The easier Fontaine stages are:.


I: Symptom-free (asymptomatic).

II: Mild claudication (leg pain while exercising)

IIb: Moderate to severe claudication.

III: Ischemic rest pain (pain in your legs when you're at rest).

IV: Ulcers or gangrene.

# Recognizing the Risk Factors

Recognizing the risk factors associated with Peripheral Artery Disease (PAD) is essential for early detection and prevention. PAD risk factors can be divided into two categories: non-modifiable and modifiable.

## Non-Modifiable Risk Factors:

**Age:** The risk of PAD increases with age, especially in individuals over 50.

**Gender:** Men are more likely to develop PAD than women, although the gender gap is narrowing.

**Family History:** If you have a family history of PAD or cardiovascular diseases, your risk may be higher.

# Modifiable Risk Factors:

**Smoking:** Smoking is one of the most significant risk factors for PAD. It not only increases the risk but also accelerates the progression of the disease.

**High Blood Pressure (Hypertension):** Uncontrolled hypertension can damage blood vessels, increasing the risk of PAD.

**High Cholesterol (Dyslipidemia):** Elevated levels of cholesterol can lead to the buildup of plaque in the arteries (ather osclerosis), narrowing blood vessels and raising the risk of PAD.

**Diabetes:** Individuals with diabetes have a higher risk of PAD due to elevated blood sugar levels that can damage blood vessels and nerves.

**Obesity:** Being overweight or obese increases the risk of PAD, as it places additional stress on the circulatory system.

**Lack of Physical Activity:** A sedentary lifestyle contributes to poor circulation and raises the risk of PAD.

**Unhealthy Diet:** Diets high in saturated fats, trans fats, and processed foods can lead to atherosclerosis and increase the risk of PAD.

**Metabolic Syndrome:** A combination of factors like obesity, high blood pressure, and high blood sugar can elevate the risk of PAD.

**High C-Reactive Protein (CRP) Levels:** Elevated levels of CRP, a marker of inflammation, are associated with an increased risk of atherosclerosis and PAD.

**Sleep Apnea:** Untreated sleep apnea can contribute to cardiovascular problems, including PAD.

**Stress**: Chronic stress can impact overall health and increase the risk of developing PAD.

Recognizing these risk factors is the first step in preventing or managing PAD. Individuals with multiple risk factors should consider lifestyle modifications and regular check-ups with a healthcare provider to assess their vascular health and take preventive measures.

# The Importance of Early Detection

The importance of early detection of Peripheral Artery Disease (PAD) cannot be overstated. Detecting PAD in its early stages can have a profound impact on an individual's health and quality of life. Here are some key reasons why early detection is crucial:

**Prevention of Complications:** Early detection allows for timely intervention and management. This can help prevent or slow down the progression of PAD, reducing the risk of severe complications such as limb amputation, heart attack, or stroke.

**Improved Quality of Life:** PAD can cause symptoms like leg pain, cramping, and difficulty walking. Identifying the condition early means that appropriate treatments and lifestyle changes can be initiated to alleviate these symptoms and improve daily functioning.

**Cardiovascular Risk Assessment**: PAD is a strong indicator of systemic atherosclerosis, a condition that affects arteries throughout the body. Detecting PAD often prompts healthcare providers to assess an individual's overall cardiovascular health, leading to the early detection of other heart-related conditions.

**Effective Management:** Early detection enables healthcare providers to tailor treatment plans to the specific needs of the individual. This may include medications, lifestyle modifications, exercise programs, and dietary changes aimed at improving blood flow and preventing further arterial damage.

**Reduced Healthcare Costs:** Managing advanced stages of PAD and its complications can be costly. Early detection and intervention can potentially reduce the financial burden on individuals and healthcare systems by preventing costly surgeries and hospitalizations.

**Increased Longevity:** Addressing PAD early can extend an individual's lifespan and enhance their overall well-being. Managing risk factors and making lifestyle changes can lead to a longer, healthier life.

**Enhanced Awareness**: Early detection raises awareness about PAD and its risk factors, prompting individuals to adopt healthier lifestyles and seek medical advice sooner if they experience symptoms.

**Preventing Critical Limb Ischemia**: In advanced cases, PAD can lead to critical limb ischemia, a severe condition where blood flow to the limbs is severely compromised. Early detection and treatment can prevent this devastating outcome.

# Chapter 2

## Navigating the Diagnostic Process

## Initial Symptoms and Warning Signs

Peripheral Artery Disease (PAD) often develops gradually, and its early symptoms can be subtle. However, recognizing these initial signs and seeking medical attention is crucial for early diagnosis and effective management. Here are some common warning signs and symptoms of PAD:

**Leg Pain:** One of the hallmark symptoms of PAD is pain, cramping, or discomfort in the legs, especially during physical activity like walking or climbing stairs. This pain, known as claudication, typically occurs in the calf muscles but can also affect the thighs or buttocks.

**Intermittent Claudication:** The pain in the legs often follows a pattern of coming and going, usually triggered by exercise or physical exertion. It tends to subside with rest.

**Numbness or Weakness:** Some individuals with PAD may experience numbness or weakness in the legs, making it difficult to walk or maintain balance.

**Coldness or Discoloration:** Reduced blood flow to the legs can lead to a sensation of coldness in the affected limb. The skin may also appear pale or bluish in color.

**Slow Hair and Nail Growth:** Slower hair and nail growth on the legs or feet can be indicative of poor blood circulation in the affected area. Sores or Wounds that Heal Slowly: PAD can impair the body's ability to heal, leading to the development of sores or wounds on the legs or feet that take a long time to heal. In severe cases, these wounds may become non-healing ulcers.

**Shiny Skin:** The skin on the legs may appear shiny and thin due to decreased blood flow. Weak or Absent Pulse: Healthcare providers often check for weakened or absent pulses in the legs or feet as part of a physical examination.

**Erectile Dysfunction:** In men, PAD can lead to erectile dysfunction (impotence) due to reduced blood flow to the genital area.

It's important to note that some individuals with PAD may not experience noticeable symptoms, especially in the early stages. This makes regular health check-ups and awareness of risk factors (such as smoking, diabetes, high blood pressure, and high cholesterol) particularly important.

Peripheral vascular disease affects 50% of patients without any symptoms. Over a lifetime, PAD might deteriorate. Sometimes symptoms don't show up until much later in life. Many people don't experience symptoms until their artery has shrunk by 60% or more.

If you experience PAD symptoms, consult a medical professional so that treatment can begin right away. It's critical to identify PAD early so that you can start the appropriate therapies before the condition worsens and causes consequences like a heart attack or stroke.

## What side effects might peripheral artery disease cause

Without therapy, persons with PAD may require an amputation, which involves cutting off all or a portion of their foot, leg, or arm (rarely both), especially if they also have diabetes.

The consequences of PAD can spread past the leg that is damaged because of how interrelated your body's circulatory system is.

Those who have atherosclerosis in their legs frequently have it elsewhere on their body.

## The Role of Medical History

The role of a comprehensive medical history in diagnosing and managing Peripheral Artery Disease (PAD) is crucial. A patient's medical history provides essential information that helps healthcare providers understand the context, potential risk factors, and nuances of their condition. Here are some key aspects of the role of medical history in PAD:

**Risk Assessment:** Medical history allows healthcare providers to assess a patient's risk factors for PAD. Information about smoking history, family history of vascular diseases, diabetes, high blood pressure, high cholesterol, and cardiovascular conditions can help identify individuals who are at higher risk of developing PAD.

**Symptom Evaluation:** A detailed medical history can reveal any symptoms or discomfort the patient is experiencing. Information about leg pain, cramping, numbness, or other symptoms associated with PAD is vital for diagnosis and determining the severity of the condition.

**Lifestyle Factors:** Understanding a patient's lifestyle is important, as habits like smoking, a sedentary lifestyle, and an unhealthy diet can contribute to the development and progression of PAD. Lifestyle modifications are a crucial component of PAD management.

**Medication and Health History:** Healthcare providers need to know about any existing medical conditions and medications the patient is taking. Certain medications, like those for blood pressure or diabetes, may be relevant in managing PAD. Additionally, underlying health conditions may interact with PAD and influence treatment decisions.

**Past Vascular Procedures:** A history of previous vascular procedures or surgeries, such as angioplasty or stent placement, can provide insights into the patient's vascular health and guide treatment choices.

**Progression of Symptoms:** For patients already diagnosed with PAD, tracking the progression of symptoms is essential. This information helps healthcare providers determine the effectiveness of current treatments and make adjustments as needed.

**Coexisting Conditions:** PAD often coexists with other cardiovascular conditions, such as coronary artery disease or carotid artery disease. A thorough medical history can identify these coexisting conditions, allowing for a comprehensive approach to treatment.

**Patient Goals and Preferences:** Understanding a patient's goals and preferences is crucial for shared decision-making in PAD management. It helps tailor treatment plans to align with the patient's values and preferences, ensuring a more patient-centered approach to care.

**Risk of Complications:** Assessing the patient's risk of complications associated with PAD, such as critical limb ischemia or non-healing ulcers, is important. This helps in planning interventions and preventative measures to minimize these risks.

**Psychosocial Factors:** A patient's medical history can provide insights into psychosocial factors that may affect their PAD management. For example, stress, anxiety, and depression can impact a patient's adherence to treatment plans, and addressing these issues may be essential.

# Diagnostic Tests and Imaging

Diagnostic tests and imaging play a vital role in confirming the presence of Peripheral Artery Disease (PAD) and assessing its severity.

Healthcare providers may use a combination of these tests to diagnose and evaluate PAD:

**Ankle-Brachial Index (ABI):** ABI is a simple and non-invasive test that measures the blood pressure in the arms and legs. A lower ABI value in the legs compared to the arms can indicate reduced blood flow and suggest PAD.

**Doppler Ultrasound**: Doppler ultrasound uses sound waves to create images of blood flow through the arteries. It can identify blockages and assess blood flow in the affected limb. Segmental Pressure Measurements: Similar to ABI, segmental pressure measurements involve taking blood pressure readings at various points along the leg to identify areas with reduced blood flow.

**Pulse Volume Recordings (PVR):** PVR is a test that measures blood volume changes in the arteries of the legs when they are compressed. It can help assess the severity and location of arterial blockages.

**Duplex Ultrasound**: Duplex ultrasound combines traditional ultrasound with Doppler technology to provide detailed images of the arteries' structure and blood flow. It is particularly useful for identifying the location and extent of blockages.

**Computed Tomography Angiography (CTA):** CTA uses a special dye and X-rays to create detailed cross-sectional images of the blood vessels. It can visualize the arteries' structure and identify blockages.

**Magnetic Resonance Angiography (MRA):** MRA uses magnetic fields and radio waves to create images of the blood vessels. It provides detailed images without the use of ionizing radiation.

**Angiography**: Angiography is an invasive procedure in which a contrast dye is injected into the arteries, followed by X-ray imaging. It can provide highly detailed images of the arteries and is often used for treatment planning.

**Toe-Brachial Index (TBI):** TBI measures the blood pressure in the toes and compares it to the blood pressure in the arms. It is particularly useful in cases where the ankle-brachial index cannot be obtained accurately.

**CT Angiography (CTA) with 3D Reconstruction:** This advanced imaging technique combines CTA with three-dimensional reconstruction to provide detailed, three-dimensional images of the arteries, aiding in treatment planning.

**Magnetic Resonance Imaging (MRI):** MRI can provide detailed images of the arteries without the use of ionizing radiation. It is useful for assessing blood flow and vessel structure.

# Chapter 3

## Lifestyle as a Foundation

### The Power of Lifestyle Modifications

Lifestyle modifications are a powerful and essential component of managing Peripheral Artery Disease (PAD). These changes can significantly improve blood flow, reduce symptoms, enhance overall vascular health, and increase the quality of life for individuals with PAD. Here's a closer look at the power of lifestyle modifications:

**Smoking Cessation:** Quitting smoking is perhaps the most impactful lifestyle change for individuals with PAD. Smoking damages blood vessels and exacerbates arterial narrowing. Quitting smoking not only slows the progression of PAD but can also improve symptoms and reduce the risk of complications.

**Regular Exercise:** Exercise is a cornerstone of PAD management. It helps improve circulation, build collateral blood vessels, and increase walking distance without pain. Structured exercise programs, such as supervised walking, can be tailored to an individual's ability and gradually increased over time.

**Healthy Diet**: Adopting a heart-healthy diet can reduce cholesterol levels, lower blood pressure, and promote overall vascular health. Emphasize a diet rich in fruits, vegetables, whole grains, lean proteins, and low-fat dairy while minimizing saturated and trans fats, salt, and sugar.

**Weight Management:** Maintaining a healthy weight or achieving weight loss if overweight can reduce the strain on the circulatory system and improve symptoms. Even modest weight loss can lead to significant benefits.

**Medication Adherence:** If prescribed medications to manage conditions like high blood pressure, high cholesterol, or diabetes, adhering to the recommended medication regimen is crucial. These medications help control risk factors for PAD and reduce complications.

**Stress Reduction:** Chronic stress can exacerbate PAD symptoms. Stress management techniques such as relaxation exercises, mindfulness, and meditation can help improve emotional well-being and potentially alleviate symptoms.

**Foot Care:** Proper foot care is vital for individuals with PAD, as they are at increased risk of foot problems and non-healing ulcers. Regular foot checks and appropriate footwear can prevent complications.

**Blood Sugar Control:** For individuals with diabetes, maintaining stable blood sugar levels is essential. Good glycemic control can slow the progression of PAD and reduce complications.

**Limiting Alcohol Consumption:** Excessive alcohol intake can contribute to high blood pressure and other cardiovascular issues. Moderation or abstinence may be advisable, depending on individual circumstances.

Medication Adjustment: Discussing PAD with a healthcare provider may lead to adjustments in medications to target specific symptoms or risk factors. Medications may be prescribed to alleviate leg pain or improve walking distance.

## Crafting a Heart-Healthy Diet

Crafting a heart-healthy diet is a fundamental component of managing Peripheral Artery Disease (PAD). A well-balanced diet can improve blood flow, reduce inflammation, lower cholesterol levels, and enhance overall vascular health. Here are guidelines for crafting a heart-healthy diet for PAD:

**Emphasize Fruits and Vegetables:**
Aim to fill half your plate with colorful fruits and vegetables. These are rich in vitamins, antioxidants, and fiber, which promote vascular health.
Berries, citrus fruits, leafy greens, and cruciferous vegetables like broccoli and Brussels sprouts are particularly beneficial.

**Choose Whole Grains:**
Opt for whole grains over refined grains. Whole grains like whole wheat, oats, quinoa, and brown rice provide fiber and nutrients that support heart health.
Avoid or limit white bread, white rice, and sugary cereals.

**Include Lean Proteins:**
Incorporate lean sources of protein such as skinless poultry, fish (especially fatty fish like salmon and mackerel), beans, lentils, and tofu. Limit red meat consumption, and when you do eat it, choose lean cuts.

**Healthy Fats:**
Focus on unsaturated fats, which can help lower cholesterol levels. Sources include olive oil, avocados, nuts, and seeds.
Limit saturated fats found in red meat, full-fat dairy products, and processed foods. Avoid trans fats entirely.

**Watch Your Sodium Intake:**
Limit salt intake to reduce high blood pressure. Use herbs, spices, and lemon juice for flavor instead of excessive salt.
Avoid highly processed and salty foods like canned soups, chips, and processed meats.
Control Portion Sizes:
Be mindful of portion sizes to avoid overeating. Smaller, more frequent meals can help maintain stable blood sugar levels and energy.

**Limit Added Sugars:**
Minimize consumption of sugary beverages, desserts, and sweets. Added sugars can contribute to inflammation and weight gain. Read food labels to identify hidden sugars in processed foods.

**Stay Hydrated:**
Drink plenty of water throughout the day.
Proper hydration is essential for overall health
and circulation.

**Moderate Alcohol Intake:**
If you choose to consume alcohol, do so in
moderation. Limit alcoholic beverages to one
drink per day for women and up to two drinks
per day for men.

**Consider Supplements:**
Talk to your healthcare provider about
appropriate supplements, such as omega-3
fatty acids or specific vitamins, to support
vascular health.

**Meal Planning:**
Plan balanced meals that incorporate a variety
of foods from different food groups.
Consider working with a registered dietitian for
personalized dietary guidance and meal
planning.

**Monitor Blood Sugar:** For individuals with
diabetes, monitoring blood sugar levels and

maintaining stable glucose levels is crucial for managing PAD.

Remember that dietary changes should be gradual and sustainable.

# Exercise and Physical Activity

Exercise and physical activity are integral components of managing Peripheral Artery Disease (PAD). A structured exercise program can improve blood flow, alleviate symptoms, and enhance the overall quality of life for individuals with PAD. Here's a guide to exercise and physical activity for PAD:

**Consult Your Healthcare Provider:** Before starting any exercise program, consult your healthcare provider, especially if you have advanced PAD or other medical conditions.

They can help determine the appropriate exercise plan for your specific needs and limitations.

**Choose Low-Impact Activities:** Low-impact exercises are gentle on the joints and less likely to cause discomfort. Consider activities like walking, stationary cycling, and swimming. These exercises promote circulation without placing excessive stress on the legs.

**Warm-Up and Cool Down:** Begin each exercise session with a 5-10 minute warm-up to gradually increase blood flow and prepare your muscles. After your workout, cool down with gentle stretches to improve flexibility and reduce muscle tension.

**Set Realistic Goals:** Establish achievable exercise goals that take your current fitness level into account. Gradually increase the duration and intensity of your workouts over time.

**Interval Training:** Some individuals with PAD benefit from interval training, where you alternate between short bursts of higher-intensity exercise and periods of lower intensity or rest. This approach can help improve walking distance and cardiovascular fitness.

**Strength Training:** Incorporate strength training exercises to build muscle. Strong leg muscles can assist with walking and reduce the effort required, potentially decreasing symptoms like leg pain.

**Monitor Symptoms:** Pay attention to any symptoms during exercise, such as leg pain or cramping. If you experience discomfort, stop and rest. Resume activity when the pain subsides.

**Walking Programs:** Walking is an excellent exercise for PAD. Start with short walks and gradually increase the duration and pace as tolerated. Walking programs, both supervised and unsupervised, can be effective in improving symptoms.

**Supervised Exercise Programs:** Consider enrolling in a supervised exercise program designed for individuals with PAD. These programs provide structured, monitored workouts tailored to your needs and abilities.

**Consistency is Key:** Aim for regular exercise. Consistency in your routine is essential for maintaining and improving vascular health. Aim for at least 150 minutes of moderate-intensity exercise per week.

**Supportive Footwear:** Wear comfortable, well-fitting shoes with cushioned soles and good arch support to reduce the risk of foot issues during exercise.

**Stay Hydrated:** Drink plenty of water before, during, and after exercise to stay properly hydrated.

**Lifestyle Integration:** Incorporate physical activity into your daily routine. For example, take short walks after meals or use a stationary bike while watching TV.

**Listen to Your Body:** If you experience severe pain, shortness of breath, or any other concerning symptoms during exercise, stop immediately and seek medical attention.

Exercise and physical activity can improve circulation, increase walking distance without pain, and enhance overall cardiovascular health for individuals with PAD.

# Smoking Cessation

Smoking cessation is one of the most critical steps individuals with Peripheral Artery Disease (PAD) can take to improve their vascular health and overall well-being. Smoking is a major risk factor for PAD, and quitting smoking can significantly slow the progression of the disease and reduce the risk of complications. Here's why smoking cessation is crucial for PAD:

**Reduced Progression of PAD:** Smoking damages blood vessels and accelerates the build-up of arterial plaque (atherosclerosis). By quitting smoking, individuals can slow down the progression of PAD, potentially preventing further narrowing of the arteries.

**Improved Blood Circulation:** Smoking constricts blood vessels and reduces blood flow, which exacerbates symptoms like leg pain and cramping in individuals with PAD. Quitting smoking can lead to improved circulation, reducing discomfort during physical activity.

**Lowered Risk of Complications:** Smoking increases the risk of complications associated with PAD, such as critical limb ischemia (severe blockage of blood flow) and non-healing ulcers. Quitting smoking can reduce the likelihood of these complications and the need for invasive treatments.

**Enhanced Response to Treatment:** Smoking can diminish the effectiveness of medications and surgical interventions used to manage PAD. By quitting smoking, individuals may respond better to treatment and experience more positive outcomes.

**Reduced Risk of Heart-Related Events:** PAD is often an indicator of systemic atherosclerosis, which affects arteries throughout the body, including those supplying the heart and brain. Quitting smoking can reduce the risk of heart attacks and strokes.

**Improved Quality of Life:** Smoking cessation can lead to improved lung function and overall physical fitness. This can result in a better quality of life for individuals with PAD, as they can engage in physical activities with less discomfort.

**Longer Life Expectancy:** Quitting smoking is associated with a longer life expectancy and improved overall health. It can reduce the risk of premature death related to cardiovascular diseases.

**Financial Savings:** Smoking is an expensive habit. By quitting, individuals can save a significant amount of money that would otherwise be spent on cigarettes.

Effective smoking cessation strategies may include:
Nicotine replacement therapy (such as nicotine gum, patches, or lozenges)
Prescription medications (such as bupropion or varenicline)
Behavioral counseling or support groups
Support from family and friends
Lifestyle changes to avoid triggers and build healthy habits
Quitting smoking can be challenging, but it is a life-changing step for individuals with PAD. It's never too late to quit

# Stress Management and Emotional Well-being

Stress management and emotional well-being play a significant role in managing Peripheral Artery Disease (PAD). The emotional impact of living with a chronic condition like PAD can be substantial, and learning to cope with stress and maintain emotional well-being is essential for overall health and symptom management. Here are some strategies for managing stress and promoting emotional well-being when living with PAD:

Educate Yourself: Understanding PAD, its causes, and its management can reduce uncertainty and anxiety. Ask your healthcare provider for information and resources to help you learn more about the condition.

Seek Support: Don't hesitate to reach out to friends, family members, or support groups. Sharing your experiences and feelings with others who understand what you're going through can provide emotional support and reduce feelings of isolation.

**Mindfulness and Relaxation Techniques:**
Mindfulness meditation, deep breathing exercises, progressive muscle relaxation, and other relaxation techniques can help reduce stress and anxiety. These practices can be integrated into your daily routine.

**Stay Active**: Regular physical activity, tailored to your capabilities, can release endorphins, which are natural mood lifters. Exercise is also beneficial for improving circulation and managing PAD symptoms.

**Set Realistic Goals:** Establish achievable goals for yourself. Celebrate small victories, whether it's walking a little farther without pain or making positive lifestyle changes.

**Balanced Lifestyle**: Maintain a balanced lifestyle that includes adequate sleep, a healthy diet, regular exercise, and stress management. Prioritize self-care to support overall well-being.

**Stay Informed**: Keep up with the latest developments in PAD research and treatment options. Being informed can empower you and reduce anxiety about the condition.

**Professional Help:** If you find that stress, anxiety, or depression is significantly affecting your quality of life, consider seeking help from a mental health professional. They can provide strategies and support tailored to your emotional well-being.

**Express Yourself:** Don't hesitate to express your feelings, fears, and concerns to your healthcare provider. They can offer guidance and connect you with resources to address emotional health.

**Limit Negative Self-Talk:** Challenge negative thoughts and self-criticism. Focus on your strengths and accomplishments, and be kind to yourself.

**Social Engagement:** Engage in social activities and maintain connections with loved ones. A strong support system can help you cope with the emotional challenges of PAD.

**Volunteer and Help Others:** Helping others can boost your sense of purpose and self-esteem. Consider volunteering or providing support to others in similar situations.

**Stay Positive:** Cultivate a positive mindset. Focus on the aspects of life that bring you joy and fulfillment.

Managing stress and promoting emotional well-being is an ongoing process. It's important to tailor these strategies to your individual needs and preferences.

# Chapter 4

## Medications and Treatment Options

## Medications to Improve Blood Flow

Medications to improve blood flow are often prescribed as part of the treatment plan for Peripheral Artery Disease (PAD). These medications aim to dilate blood vessels, reduce blood clot formation, and improve circulation in the affected limbs. Here are some common medications used to improve blood flow for PAD:

### Antiplatelet Agents:

**Aspirin**: Low-dose aspirin is often prescribed to reduce the risk of blood clot formation. It helps prevent platelets from clumping together, improving blood flow.

**Clopidogrel (Plavix):** This antiplatelet medication is an alternative to aspirin and may be prescribed in cases of aspirin intolerance or as an adjunct therapy.

Anticoagulants:

**Warfarin (Coumadin):** Warfarin is an anticoagulant that can help prevent blood clots from forming in the arteries. It may be prescribed in cases where there is a higher risk of clot formation.

**Statins:**

Atorvastatin (Lipitor), Rosuvastatin (Crestor), Simvastatin (Zocor), etc.: Statins are prescribed to lower cholesterol levels. By reducing the buildup of plaque in the arteries, they can improve blood flow and reduce the risk of atherosclerosis-related complications.

**Cilostazol (Pletal):** Cilostazol is a medication specifically approved for treating the symptoms of intermittent claudication associated with

PAD. It works by dilating blood vessels and reducing blood viscosity, which can improve walking distance without pain.

**Pentoxifylline (Trental):** Pentoxifylline is another medication used to improve blood flow in individuals with PAD. It helps make red blood cells more flexible, enhancing circulation.

**ACE Inhibitors and ARBs:** These medications, such as Enalapril (Vasotec) or Losartan (Cozaar), are typically prescribed for individuals with high blood pressure. They can help relax blood vessels and improve blood flow.

**Vasodilators**: Certain vasodilator medications, like nitrates (nitroglycerin), can help dilate blood vessels temporarily, which can provide relief from symptoms like leg pain and improve blood flow.

Medications to Control Diabetes and Blood **Pressure**: For individuals with PAD who also have diabetes or high blood pressure, medications to manage these conditions are crucial. Better control of these risk factors can improve blood flow and reduce PAD symptoms.

**Chelation Therapy**: Some individuals may explore chelation therapy, which involves the use of intravenous medications to remove heavy metals from the bloodstream. It is considered an alternative therapy and should be discussed with a healthcare provider.

It's important to note that medication choices and dosages will be determined by your healthcare provider based on your specific PAD symptoms, risk factors, and overall health.

# Blood Thinners and Antiplatelet Agents

commonly prescribed medications for individuals with Peripheral Artery Disease (PAD) to reduce the risk of blood clots and improve blood flow. These medications work by preventing excessive clot formation in the arteries affected by PAD. Here's an overview of blood thinners and antiplatelet agents used in PAD management:

**Aspirin**: Low-dose aspirin is one of the most widely prescribed antiplatelet agents for PAD. It inhibits platelets from clumping together, reducing the risk of clot formation in the arteries. Aspirin is often the initial choice due to its effectiveness and affordability.

**Clopidogrel (Plavix):** Clopidogrel is another antiplatelet medication used to prevent blood clot formation. It is often prescribed as an alternative or in combination with aspirin, especially for individuals who are intolerant to aspirin.

**Ticagrelor (Brilinta) and Prasugrel (Effient):** These are newer antiplatelet medications that may be used in specific cases, typically in individuals with a history of coronary artery disease or those who have undergone procedures like stent placement. They work by blocking platelets more effectively than aspirin.

**Warfarin (Coumadin):** Warfarin is an anticoagulant medication that inhibits blood clot formation by interfering with the body's clotting factors. It is used in certain situations where there is a higher risk of clot formation. Regular monitoring of blood clotting times (INR) is necessary when taking warfarin.
Rivaroxaban (Xarelto), Apixaban (Eliquis), and

**Dabigatran (Pradaxa):** These are newer oral anticoagulant medications that are sometimes considered for PAD management in specific cases. They have advantages over warfarin as they do not require frequent blood monitoring.

**Cilostazol (Pletal):** While not a blood thinner or antiplatelet agent in the traditional sense, cilostazol is a medication specifically approved for improving symptoms of intermittent claudication in PAD. It works by dilating blood vessels and inhibiting platelet aggregation.

It's important to note that the choice of medication and the specific regimen will depend on the individual's overall health, risk factors, and the severity of PAD. Your healthcare provider will carefully evaluate your condition and prescribe the most appropriate medication or combination of medications to manage your PAD effectively.

As with any medication, it's essential to take these drugs as prescribed and to adhere to the recommended treatment plan.

# Minimally Invasive Procedures

Blood thinners and antiplatelet agents are commonly prescribed medications for individuals with Peripheral Artery Disease (PAD) to reduce the risk of blood clots and improve blood flow. These medications work by preventing excessive clot formation in the arteries affected by PAD. Here's an overview of blood thinners and antiplatelet agents used in PAD management:

**Aspirin**: Low-dose aspirin is one of the most widely prescribed antiplatelet agents for PAD. It inhibits platelets from clumping together, reducing the risk of clot formation in the arteries. Aspirin is often the initial choice due to its effectiveness and affordability.

**Clopidogrel (Plavix):** Clopidogrel is another antiplatelet medication used to prevent blood clot formation. It is often prescribed as an alternative or in combination with aspirin, especially for individuals who are intolerant to aspirin.

**Ticagrelor (Brilinta) and Prasugrel (Effient):** These are newer antiplatelet medications that may be used in specific cases, typically in individuals with a history of coronary artery disease or those who have undergone procedures like stent placement. They work by blocking platelets more effectively than aspirin.

**Warfarin (Coumadin):** Warfarin is an anticoagulant medication that inhibits blood clot formation by interfering with the body's clotting factors. It is used in certain situations where there is a higher risk of clot formation. Regular monitoring of blood clotting times (INR) is necessary when taking warfarin.
Rivaroxaban (Xarelto), Apixaban (Eliquis), and

**Dabigatran (Pradaxa):** These are newer oral anticoagulant medications that are sometimes considered for PAD management in specific cases. They have advantages over warfarin as they do not require frequent blood monitoring.

**Cilostazol (Pletal):** While not a blood thinner or antiplatelet agent in the traditional sense, cilostazol is a medication specifically approved for improving symptoms of intermittent claudication in PAD. It works by dilating blood vessels and inhibiting platelet aggregation.

It's important to note that the choice of medication and the specific regimen will depend on the individual's overall health, risk factors, and the severity of PAD. Your healthcare provider will carefully evaluate your condition and prescribe the most appropriate medication or combination of medications to manage your PAD effectively.

# Surgical Interventions

Surgical interventions may be necessary for individuals with Peripheral Artery Disease (PAD) when minimally invasive procedures and conservative treatments are not sufficient to improve blood flow or manage complications. Surgical options aim to restore blood flow to the affected areas and reduce the risk of complications. Here are some common surgical interventions for PAD:

Bypass Grafting: In bypass grafting, a surgeon creates a detour around the blocked or narrowed artery by using a graft (a blood vessel or synthetic tube). This graft allows blood to flow around the obstruction and reach the target area, restoring blood flow. Common types of bypass grafting include:

- **Aortobifemoral Bypass:** Used to bypass blockages in the aorta and femoral arteries.
- **Femoropopliteal Bypass:** Performed to bypass blockages in the femoral artery,

often extending down to the popliteal artery.

**Endarterectomy**: Endarterectomy is a surgical procedure that involves the removal of plaque from the inner lining of the affected artery. It is often used in larger arteries and may be performed in the carotid arteries (carotid endarterectomy) or the aorta (aortic endarterectomy). By clearing the blockage, endarterectomy improves blood flow.

**Thromboendarterectomy**: This surgical procedure is performed when there is a blood clot (thrombus) in an artery. The surgeon removes both the clot and any underlying plaque to restore blood flow. It is typically used in emergencies when there is a severe blockage or acute limb-threatening ischemia.

**Angioplasty with Stent Placement (Surgical Bypass Alternative)**: In some cases, when minimally invasive angioplasty is not possible or not successful, surgical bypass may be considered. This involves creating a bypass graft to redirect blood flow around the blocked artery, similar to endovascular stenting procedures.

**Limb Amputation:** In severe cases where PAD has led to extensive tissue damage, non-healing ulcers, or gangrene, amputation may be necessary to remove the affected tissue and prevent the spread of infection. The goal is to preserve as much healthy tissue as possible while improving overall health and mobility.

Surgical interventions for PAD are typically considered when there is a high risk of limb loss, severe pain, or life-threatening complications. These procedures are often performed by vascular surgeons with expertise in treating PAD. The choice of surgery depends on the location and severity of the blockage, the patient's overall health, and individual circumstances.

Recovery from surgical interventions may require a hospital stay and post-operative rehabilitation to regain mobility and function.

# Chapter 5

## Your Journey to Recovery

# Setting Realistic Goals

Setting realistic goals is an important aspect of effectively managing Peripheral Artery Disease (PAD). Realistic goals help individuals with PAD focus on achievable outcomes, monitor progress, and stay motivated to make positive lifestyle changes. Here are some guidelines for setting realistic goals in the fight against PAD:

**Consult with Healthcare Providers:** Start by discussing your goals with your healthcare provider, such as a vascular specialist or cardiologist. They can provide guidance on what is achievable given your specific condition, overall health, and any limitations.
**Understand Your Condition**: Gain a clear understanding of your PAD, including the severity of your arterial blockages and your current symptoms. This knowledge will help you set goals that align with your unique situation.
**Prioritize Goals:** Determine which aspects of your health and well-being are most important to you. These priorities may include reducing leg pain, increasing walking distance, quitting smoking, managing diabetes

or hypertension, or improving overall cardiovascular health.

**Start Small:** Begin with small, achievable goals that can be easily integrated into your daily routine. For example, if you're currently sedentary, your initial goal might be to take short walks several times a week.

**Be Specific and Measurable:** Define your goals in specific and measurable terms. For example, rather than setting a vague goal like "I want to improve my walking," specify that you aim to walk for 10 minutes without pain.

**Set Incremental Targets:** Break larger goals into smaller, manageable milestones. This allows you to celebrate progress along the way. For instance, if your long-term goal is to walk a mile without pain, set intermediate goals to reach specific distances first.

**Consider Timeframes:** Establish realistic timeframes for achieving your goals. Be patient with yourself and recognize that progress may take time. For example, you might aim to increase your walking distance by 10% each month.

**Seek Support:** Share your goals with friends and family members who can provide encouragement and accountability. Consider joining a support group for individuals with PAD.

**Track Progress:** Keep a record of your progress. This could involve maintaining a journal of your activities, tracking your walking distances, or monitoring your medication adherence.

**Stay Flexible:** Be willing to adjust your goals as needed based on your health status and any changes in your condition. Sometimes, goals may need to be adapted to new circumstances.

**Celebrate Achievements:** Celebrate your successes, no matter how small they may seem. Acknowledging your achievements can boost motivation and confidence.

**Stay Informed:** Continue to educate yourself about PAD, its management, and treatment options. Knowledge empowers you to make informed decisions and set relevant goals.

**Regular Check-Ins:** Schedule regular follow-up appointments with your healthcare provider to discuss your progress, adjust your treatment plan, and refine your goals as necessary.

Remember that the fight against PAD is a journey, and setting realistic goals is a key part of that journey. By focusing on achievable objectives, individuals with PAD can improve their quality of life and work towards better vascular health.

# Tracking Your Progress

Tracking your progress when managing Peripheral Artery Disease (PAD) is crucial for monitoring the effectiveness of your treatment plan and making informed decisions about your care. Here are some key steps and strategies for tracking your progress with PAD:

**Consult Your Healthcare Provider:** Start by discussing your goals and progress-tracking strategies with your healthcare provider. They can provide guidance on the specific aspects of your condition to monitor and how frequently to do so.

**Maintain a Symptom Journal:** Keep a journal or diary to record your symptoms and their severity. Note when you experience leg pain or discomfort, the duration of symptoms, and any specific activities or circumstances that trigger or alleviate symptoms.

**Walking Distance:** Measure your walking distance regularly to assess improvements. Use landmarks or a pedometer to track how far you can walk without pain or discomfort. Gradually aim to increase this distance over time.

**Pain Assessment:** Rate your leg pain or discomfort on a scale from 0 to 10 during and after physical activities. This can help you and your healthcare provider assess changes in pain levels.

**Medication Adherence:** Keep a medication log to track when you take prescribed medications. Consistent adherence to your medication regimen is essential for managing PAD effectively.

**Blood Pressure and Other Vital Signs:** Monitor your blood pressure, heart rate, and other vital signs regularly, especially if you have hypertension or other cardiovascular conditions.

**Diet and Exercise:** Maintain a record of your dietary choices and exercise routines. Note any changes in your eating habits and physical activity levels. Tracking these factors can help you identify patterns that affect your PAD symptoms.

**Lifestyle Changes:** Record any lifestyle modifications you've implemented, such as quitting smoking, adopting a heart-healthy diet, or participating in a structured exercise program.

**Weight and Body Measurements:** Keep track of your weight and body measurements, such as waist circumference, if weight management is a part of your PAD management plan.

**Wound Care:** If you have non-healing ulcers or other skin issues related to PAD, document their progress and any changes in appearance or healing status. Photographs can be helpful for visual documentation.

**Regular Check-Ups:** Attend regular follow-up appointments with your healthcare provider. These appointments are essential for evaluating your progress, adjusting your treatment plan, and addressing any concerns.

**Use Health Apps and Devices:** Consider using health tracking apps or wearable devices to monitor your physical activity, heart rate, and other relevant metrics. Many of these tools can sync data with your healthcare provider's electronic health record system.

**Set Milestones**: Define specific milestones or goals for your PAD management, such as increasing walking distance by a certain percentage or achieving target blood pressure levels.

**Share Your Progress**: Share your progress reports with your healthcare provider during appointments. This information will help them assess the effectiveness of your treatment plan and make necessary adjustments.

Regularly tracking your progress with PAD provides valuable insights into how your condition is evolving and how well your treatment plan is working.

# Navigating Potential Setbacks

Navigating potential setbacks when managing Peripheral Artery Disease (PAD) is an important part of the journey toward improved vascular health. While progress may not always be linear, there are strategies to address setbacks and continue working towards your goals. Here's how to navigate common setbacks associated with PAD:

**Recognize That Setbacks Can Happen:**
Understand that managing a chronic condition like PAD can involve ups and downs. Setbacks

are a normal part of the process, and they don't diminish your long-term progress.

**Stay Informed:**
Continue educating yourself about PAD and its management. Knowledge empowers you to understand your condition better and make informed decisions during setbacks.

**Communicate with Your Healthcare Provider:**
If you experience a setback in symptoms or overall health, reach out to your healthcare provider promptly. They can assess the situation, adjust your treatment plan, and provide guidance on managing the setback.

**Review and Adjust Your Goals:**
If setbacks hinder your ability to achieve your goals, consider revising them to be more achievable in the short term. Focus on small, manageable steps that align with your current health status.

**Lifestyle Modifications:**

Revisit and reinforce lifestyle changes that are within your control, such as maintaining a heart-healthy diet, quitting smoking, and engaging in regular physical activity.

**Physical Activity:**
If symptoms or setbacks make it challenging to maintain your exercise routine, discuss alternative activities or modifications with your healthcare provider. You may need to adjust the frequency or intensity of exercise during particularly challenging times.

**Medication Adherence:**
Ensure you're consistently taking prescribed medications as directed. Missing doses or discontinuing medications without medical supervision can lead to setbacks.

**Stress Management:**
Implement stress-reduction techniques such as mindfulness, deep breathing exercises, or relaxation to cope with emotional challenges associated with setbacks.

**Seek Emotional Support:**
Lean on friends, family, or support groups to share your feelings and concerns during setbacks. Emotional support can make a significant difference in managing the emotional impact of PAD.

**Maintain Regular Check-Ups:**
Continue attending scheduled follow-up appointments with your healthcare provider, even during setbacks. Regular monitoring is essential for assessing your progress and making adjustments as needed.

**Adjust Expectations:**
Understand that PAD management may involve temporary limitations. Be patient with yourself and recognize that setbacks are not failures but opportunities for growth.

**Wound Care:**
If you have non-healing ulcers or wounds, diligent wound care is crucial. Seek specialized wound care if needed and follow your healthcare provider's recommendations.

**Stay Positive:**
Maintain a positive mindset and focus on your long-term goals. A positive attitude can help you overcome setbacks and stay motivated.

Remember that managing PAD is a journey, and setbacks are a natural part of that journey.

# Celebrating Small Wins

Celebrating small wins is a powerful and motivating practice, especially when managing a chronic condition like Peripheral Artery Disease (PAD). Recognizing and celebrating even the smallest achievements can boost your morale, reinforce positive habits, and provide motivation to continue your journey toward better vascular health. Here's how to celebrate small wins in your battle against PAD:

**Set Clear Milestones:** Define clear, achievable milestones related to your PAD management. These milestones should be specific, measurable, and realistic. For example, a milestone could be walking a certain distance without experiencing pain.

**Acknowledge Progress**: Regularly acknowledge and celebrate your progress, no matter how small it may seem. Recognize the effort you've put into managing your condition and the positive changes you've made.

**Reward Yourself:** Consider incorporating small rewards when you reach your milestones. These rewards don't have to be extravagant; they can be simple pleasures like enjoying a favorite healthy snack, treating yourself to a relaxing bath, or watching a movie you love.

**Maintain a Journal:** Keep a journal or progress log where you record your achievements, no matter how minor. Write down the date, the milestone achieved, and any feelings or thoughts associated with it. Reflecting on your journey can be gratifying.

**Share Your Success:** Share your achievements with supportive friends, family members, or a support group. Sharing your wins with others who understand your challenges can make the celebration even more meaningful.

**Visual Reminders:** Create visual reminders of your progress. You might use a calendar to mark off successful days, create a vision board with images representing your goals, or use a mobile app to track your achievements.

**Positive Self-Talk:** Practice positive self-talk and self-encouragement. Recognize the strength and resilience you've demonstrated in managing PAD.

**Track Health Metrics:** Monitor improvements in health metrics, such as improved blood pressure, lower cholesterol levels, or better blood sugar control. These tangible improvements are worth celebrating.

**Set New Goals:** As you achieve your milestones, set new ones. Continuously challenging yourself with fresh goals keeps you engaged and motivated in your PAD management journey.

**Celebrate Healthier Habits:** Celebrate the adoption of healthier habits, whether it's eating more fruits and vegetables, reducing stress through relaxation techniques, or consistently taking prescribed medications.

**Create a Supportive Environment:** Surround yourself with a supportive environment that encourages your progress. Share your achievements with friends and family who can offer encouragement.

**Stay Consistent:** Consistency in celebrating small wins is key. Regularly acknowledging your achievements can help maintain your motivation and positive momentum.

Remember that managing PAD is a long-term commitment, and each small win contributes to your overall progress.

# Chapter 6

## Beyond the Physical: Emotional Resilience

## Coping with Emotional Challenges

Coping with emotional challenges when living with Peripheral Artery Disease (PAD) is an important aspect of managing the condition effectively. PAD can have a significant impact on a person's emotional well-being due to its chronic nature and potential limitations on daily activities. Here are strategies to help you cope with emotional challenges associated with PAD:

**Educate Yourself:** Knowledge is empowering. Learn as much as you can about PAD, including its causes, symptoms, treatments, and prognosis. Understanding your condition can reduce anxiety and uncertainty.

**Open Communication:** Share your feelings and concerns with your healthcare provider. They can provide guidance, address your questions, and offer emotional support.

**Build a Support System:**
Talk to friends and family about your condition. They can provide emotional support, lend a listening ear, and offer assistance when needed.
Consider joining a support group for individuals with PAD. Sharing experiences with others who understand your challenges can be comforting.

**Manage Stress:**
Practice stress management techniques such as mindfulness, meditation, deep breathing exercises, or progressive muscle relaxation. Engage in enjoyable activities or hobbies that help you relax and take your mind off PAD-related stress.

**Set Realistic Goals:**
Set achievable goals for managing your condition. Celebrate small successes to boost your confidence and motivation.

*Certainly, here are more strategies for coping with emotional challenges associated with Peripheral Artery Disease (PAD):*

**Seek Professional Help**: If you find that emotional challenges are significantly affecting your quality of life, consider speaking with a mental health professional. They can provide strategies and support tailored to your emotional well-being.

**Express Your Feelings:** Don't hesitate to express your feelings, fears, and concerns to your healthcare provider. They can offer guidance and connect you with resources to address emotional health.

**Mindful Acceptance:** Acknowledge that living with a chronic condition like PAD can be emotionally challenging at times. Practice mindful acceptance by recognizing your feelings without judgment.

**Engage in Physical Activity:** Regular physical activity, within the limits of your condition, can release endorphins, which are natural mood lifters. Exercise can also help reduce stress and improve overall emotional well-being.

**Adapt to Limitations:** Understand that there may be limitations on certain activities due to PAD. Instead of focusing on what you can't do, shift your focus to what you can do within your capabilities.

**Maintain a Positive Mindset:** Cultivate a positive outlook by focusing on the aspects of life that bring you joy and fulfillment. Surround yourself with positivity and engage in activities that uplift your spirits.

**Stay Informed:** Keep up with the latest developments in PAD research and treatment options. Being informed can empower you and reduce anxiety about the condition.

**Social Engagement:** Engage in social activities and maintain connections with loved ones. A strong support system can help you cope with the emotional challenges of PAD.

**Volunteer and Help Others:** Helping others can boost your sense of purpose and self-esteem. Consider volunteering or providing support to others in similar situations.

**Limit Negative Self-Talk:** Challenge negative thoughts and self-criticism. Focus on your strengths and accomplishments, and be kind to yourself.

Remember that it's okay to experience a range of emotions when living with PAD.

# Coping with Emotional Challenges

Coping with emotional challenges when dealing with Peripheral Artery Disease (PAD) is essential for maintaining your overall well-being. PAD can have a significant impact on your life, both physically and emotionally. Here are specific strategies to help you cope with the emotional challenges associated with PAD:

**Seek Emotional Support:** Reach out to friends and family members for emotional support. Sharing your feelings and concerns with loved ones can provide comfort and understanding.

**Join a Support Group:** Consider joining a support group for individuals with PAD. Connecting with others who are going through similar experiences can be reassuring and offer valuable insights.

**Talk to a Mental Health Professional:** If you find that your emotional challenges are overwhelming or persistent, consider speaking with a therapist or counselor. They can provide strategies to cope with anxiety, depression, or stress related to your condition.

**Educate Yourself:** Learn more about PAD, its causes, symptoms, and treatment options. Understanding your condition can help reduce fear and uncertainty.

**Set Realistic Goals:** Establish achievable goals for managing your PAD. Celebrate small victories, such as walking a little farther without pain or making positive lifestyle changes.

**Engage in Relaxation Techniques:** Practice relaxation techniques such as deep breathing exercises, mindfulness meditation, or progressive muscle relaxation to reduce stress and anxiety.

**Stay Active Within Your Limits:** Engage in physical activity that is safe and within the limits of your condition. Regular exercise can boost mood and reduce stress.

**Express Your Feelings:** Don't hesitate to share your feelings, fears, and concerns with your healthcare provider. They can offer guidance and connect you with resources to address emotional health.

**Maintain a Positive Mindset:** Cultivate a positive outlook by focusing on the aspects of life that bring you joy and fulfillment. Surround yourself with positivity and engage in activities that uplift your spirits.

**Practice Self-Compassion:** Be kind to yourself and avoid self-blame. Living with a chronic condition like PAD is challenging, and it's important to acknowledge your efforts and resilience.

**Stay Informed:** Stay informed about the latest developments in PAD research and treatment options. Being knowledgeable about your condition can empower you and reduce anxiety.

**Social Engagement:** Continue participating in social activities and maintain connections with loved ones. A strong support system can help you cope with the emotional challenges of PAD.

**Set Realistic Expectations:** Understand that living with PAD may involve some limitations, but it doesn't define your entire life. Adjust your expectations to align with your current abilities.

**Celebrate Small Achievements:** Celebrate even small achievements and milestones in your PAD management journey. These victories, no matter how minor, deserve recognition.

## Staying Positive and Motivated

Staying positive and motivated while living with Peripheral Artery Disease (PAD) is crucial for maintaining your overall well-being and effectively managing your condition. Here are strategies to help you maintain a positive mindset and stay motivated:

**Educate Yourself**: Knowledge is empowering. Learn about PAD, its causes, symptoms, and treatment options. Understanding your condition can reduce fear and uncertainty.

**Set Clear Goals:** Establish specific, achievable goals related to your PAD management. These goals can provide motivation and a sense of purpose. Celebrate your achievements, no matter how small.

**Stay Active Within Your Limits:** Engage in regular physical activity that is safe and within your capabilities. Even small amounts of exercise can improve circulation, reduce symptoms, and boost mood.
Healthy Eating: Adopt a heart-healthy diet rich in fruits, vegetables, whole grains, lean proteins, and low in saturated fats and sodium. A well-balanced diet can support your overall health and energy levels.

**Medication Adherence:** Take prescribed medications as directed by your healthcare provider. Consistency with your medication regimen is crucial for managing PAD effectively.

**Manage Risk Factors:** Address other risk factors for PAD, such as high blood pressure, high cholesterol, and diabetes. Well-managed risk factors can improve your overall health and reduce PAD-related complications.

**Embrace a Positive Mindset:** Focus on the aspects of life that bring you joy and fulfillment. Cultivate a positive outlook by practicing gratitude and optimism.

**Stay Informed:** Stay up-to-date with the latest advancements in PAD treatment and management. Being informed can empower you and give you hope for potential improvements in your condition.

**Lean on Support:** Seek emotional support from friends, family, or a support group. Sharing your experiences and feelings with others who understand can provide comfort and encouragement.

**Manage Stress:** Practice stress-reduction techniques such as mindfulness meditation, deep breathing exercises, or progressive muscle relaxation. Stress management can positively impact your overall health.

**Visualize Your Goals:** Create a vision board or use visualization techniques to imagine yourself achieving your goals and living a fulfilling life despite PAD.

**Celebrate Small Wins:** Acknowledge and celebrate your achievements, no matter how minor. Recognizing your efforts can boost motivation and self-esteem.

**Adapt to Challenges:** Understand that managing PAD may involve challenges and setbacks. Adapt to these challenges by seeking solutions and staying resilient.

**Stay Active Socially:** Continue engaging in social activities and maintaining connections with loved ones. A strong support system can provide encouragement and motivation.

**Stay Persistent:** Consistency is key to managing PAD. Continue with your prescribed treatments, lifestyle changes, and follow-up appointments, even when faced with obstacles.

**Positive Self-Talk:** Challenge negative thoughts and practice positive self-talk. Remind yourself of your strengths and capabilities.

# 30 DAYS EXERCISE FOR YOU

Exercise can be beneficial for people with Peripheral Artery Disease (PAD) as it can improve circulation, reduce symptoms, and increase walking distance. However, it's crucial to approach exercise with caution and consult your healthcare provider before starting any new exercise routine. Here's a 30-day exercise plan designed for individuals with PAD. Please adapt it to your specific capabilities and consult your healthcare provider for personalized guidance:

## Week 1: Gentle Warm-up and Stretching

## Days 1-7:

Day 1: Start with a 5-minute gentle warm-up, like ankle pumps and seated leg lifts. Then, perform 5 minutes of stretching exercises for your legs and ankles.

Days 2-7: Gradually increase the warm-up and stretching time to 10 minutes each day.

Week 2: Low-Intensity Walking

## Days 8-14:

Days 8-14: Begin with a 10-minute warm-up and stretching session.

Start with 5 minutes of slow-paced, flat-surface walking. Pay attention to any discomfort or pain. If you experience discomfort, stop and rest.
Gradually increase your walking time by 1-2 minutes each day, but do not push yourself too hard. The goal is to build endurance gradually.
Week 3: Moderate-Intensity Walking

Days 15-21:

Days 15-21: Continue with a 10-minute warm-up and stretching session.
Increase your walking intensity to a brisk pace for 5-10 minutes, followed by a slower pace for 5 minutes.
Gradually increase your brisk walking time by 1-2 minutes each day.

Week 4: Interval Walking

Days 22-30:

Days 22-30: Start with a 10-minute warm-up and stretching session.
Incorporate interval walking: Walk briskly for 2-3 minutes, then slow down for 2-3 minutes to recover. Repeat this cycle for 20-30 minutes.
Focus on consistency and gradually increase the intensity or duration of your brisk intervals as tolerated.
Additional Tips:

Always listen to your body. If you experience pain, discomfort, or severe fatigue, stop and rest.

Pay attention to the time of day when you feel best for exercise, whether it's morning, afternoon, or evening.

Stay hydrated throughout your exercise sessions.

Choose flat and even surfaces for walking to minimize the risk of tripping or falling.

Consider walking indoors, such as at a shopping mall or fitness center, during inclement weather or extreme temperatures.

Remember that the goal of this 30-day plan is to gradually build your endurance and improve your walking capacity. It's important to consult your healthcare provider before starting or modifying any exercise routine, as they can provide personalized recommendations based on your specific condition and needs.

# 30 DAYS MEAL PLAN.

A heart-healthy meal plan is crucial for individuals with Peripheral Artery Disease (PAD) to manage their condition effectively. Here's a 30-day meal plan with ingredients and preparation tips tailored to support vascular health:

Week 1:

Day 1 - Breakfast:

Ingredients: Oatmeal with fresh berries (blueberries, strawberries) and a sprinkle of chopped nuts (almonds or walnuts).

Lunch: Grilled chicken salad with mixed greens, cherry tomatoes, cucumber, and balsamic vinaigrette.

Dinner: Baked salmon with steamed broccoli and quinoa.

Day 2 - Breakfast:

Ingredients: Greek yogurt parfait with honey, sliced banana, and granola.

Lunch: Lentil soup with a side of mixed greens and whole-grain bread.

Dinner: Grilled shrimp with roasted asparagus and brown rice.

Day 3 - Breakfast:

Ingredients: Whole-grain toast with avocado spread and poached eggs.

Lunch: Turkey and vegetable stir-fry with brown rice.

Dinner: Baked cod with sautéed spinach and quinoa.

Day 4 - Breakfast:

Ingredients: Smoothie with spinach, banana, unsweetened almond milk, and a scoop of protein powder.

Lunch: Chickpea salad with diced cucumber, red onion, parsley, and lemon-tahini dressing.

Dinner: Grilled chicken breast with roasted Brussels sprouts and sweet potato.

Day 5 - Breakfast:

Ingredients: Whole-grain waffles topped with Greek yogurt and mixed berries.

Lunch: Mixed bean and vegetable chili with a side of whole-grain crackers.
Dinner: Baked trout with sautéed kale and quinoa.
Day 6 - Breakfast:

Ingredients: Scrambled eggs with diced bell peppers and a side of whole-grain toast.
Lunch: Spinach and quinoa salad with roasted beets, goat cheese, and vinaigrette.
Dinner: Grilled tofu with steamed broccoli and brown rice.
Day 7 - Breakfast:

Ingredients: Overnight oats with chia seeds, almond milk, sliced banana, and a drizzle of honey.
Lunch: Caprese salad with fresh tomatoes, mozzarella, basil, and a balsamic glaze.

Dinner: Baked chicken breast with sautéed green beans and quinoa.

Week 2-4: Continue to vary your meals with similar heart-healthy ingredients, including lean proteins (fish, poultry, legumes), whole grains, plenty of fruits and vegetables, and healthy fats (avocado, nuts, olive oil). Limit sodium, processed foods, and saturated fats.

## Preparation Tips:

Use olive oil or canola oil for cooking.
Opt for whole grains like brown rice, quinoa, and whole-grain pasta.
Season dishes with herbs and spices instead of salt.

Include a variety of colorful fruits and vegetables to ensure a wide range of nutrients.

Choose lean protein sources like chicken, turkey, fish, tofu, and legumes.

Keep portion sizes in check to manage calorie intake.

Drink plenty of water throughout the day.

Snack on heart-healthy options like raw nuts, Greek yogurt, and fresh fruit.

Consult with a registered dietitian or healthcare provider to tailor this meal plan to your specific dietary needs and any other medical conditions you may have. They can provide personalized guidance to support your vascular health and overall well-being.

# Conclusion

In conclusion, this book on Peripheral Artery Disease (PAD) has aimed to provide you with valuable insights, practical guidance, and a roadmap to effectively manage this chronic condition. Throughout these pages, we have explored the intricacies of PAD, from its causes and risk factors to its symptoms, diagnosis, and treatment options.

We've delved into lifestyle modifications, emphasizing the significance of adopting a heart-healthy diet, staying physically active, and managing stress as key pillars of PAD management. By empowering yourself with knowledge and making informed choices, you can take control of your vascular health.

We've also touched on the importance of medication adherence, surgical interventions, and minimally invasive procedures when necessary, highlighting the collaborative relationship between you and your healthcare provider.

Remember that living with PAD is a journey, and it's natural to encounter challenges along the way. However, with dedication, a positive mindset, and the support of your healthcare team, you can effectively manage your condition, improve your quality of life, and reduce the risk of complications.

As you move forward in your PAD management journey, continue to prioritize your health, set achievable goals, and celebrate your victories, no matter how small. You have the strength and resilience to navigate this path and enjoy a fulfilling life despite the challenges posed by PAD.

Always remember that you are not alone in this journey. Lean on your support system, seek professional guidance when needed, and stay committed to your well-being. With each step you take, you're moving closer to better vascular health and a brighter future.

Thank you for choosing this book as your resource, and may your journey towards improved vascular health be filled with hope, determination, and ultimately, success.

www.ingramcontent.com/pod-product-compliance
Lightning Source LLC
Chambersburg PA
CBHW062335290526
45794CB00005B/2044